PEGAN DIET COOKBOOK

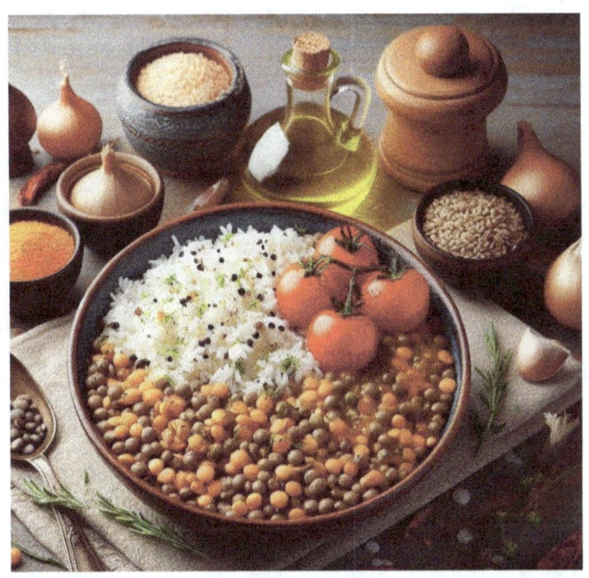

Quick and Tasty Paleo and Vegan Recipes and Meal Plan For Improved Lifelong Health

Robert Elliot

Copyright © Robert Elliot (2023)

The contents of this book are based on the author's research, knowledge, and experience. They are meant for educational purposes only and should not be taken as medical advice. Readers should consult their healthcare provider before making any changes to their health regimen.

Table of Contents

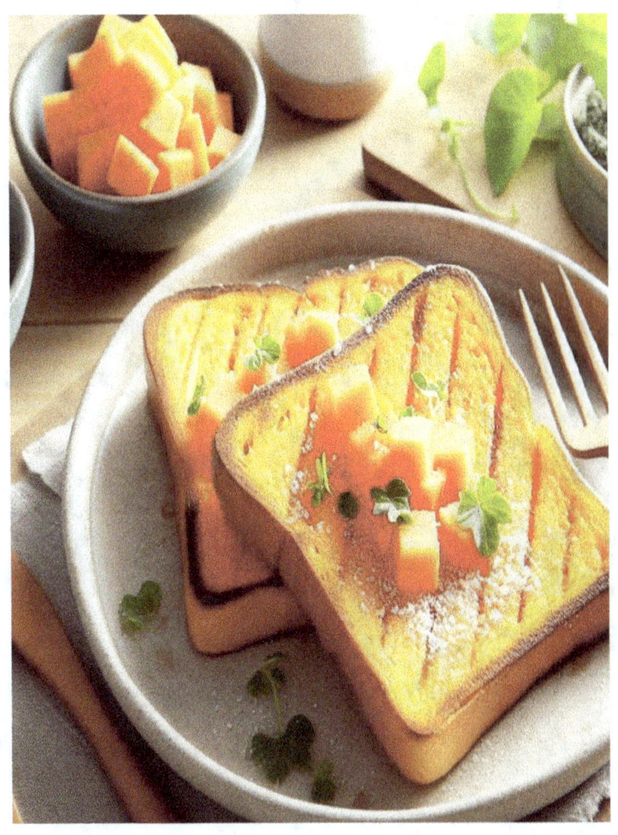

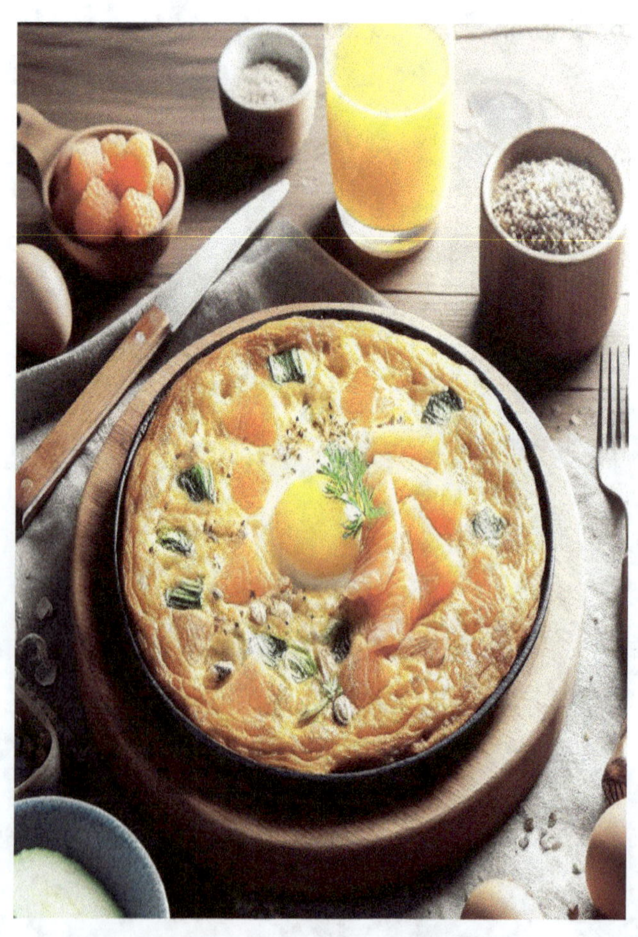

Introduction

I was still in medical school when I first heard my dad mention the Pegan Diet in passing. Honestly, it sounded like just another health gimmick. But let me tell you, that throwaway comment turned my world upside down in the most unexpected way possible.

Here I was, knee-deep in textbooks and hospital rounds, surviving on a cocktail of caffeine and takeout meals. Sound familiar? Yeah, it's the classic med student survival kit. Until one day, curiosity nudged me to give the Pegan thing a shot. Trust me; I had zero expectations.

I dove headfirst into this wild new world of eating—the Pegan way. Forget the rabbit food stereotype; this wasn't about munching on flavorless leaves. This was a culinary escapade where taste, health, and vitality collided in the most epic way possible.

Bite after bite, meal after meal, I discovered a universe where flavors danced, ingredients shone, and meals weren't just about survival but about thriving. And let me tell you, it was a revelation!

But here's the kicker: this wasn't just about the taste. Nah, it was about waking up without a foggy brain, sailing through the day without those energy nosedives, and, hold your breath, sleeping like a baby after a lullaby marathon.

I'll let you in on a secret—it's not some hocus-pocus. Nope. It's a well-crafted harmony of all things good for you. Proteins? Check. Healthy fats? Double-check. Veggies and fruits? You bet. It's a symphony of nutrients that your body craves, served up on a plate that screams, "Hey, I got you covered!"

So listen up, fellow seekers of wellness and food enthusiasts alike! The Pegan Diet Cookbook isn't just some diet recipe book; it's a game-changer. Stay tuned, and I'll show you how this delicious revolution can transform your life from "meh" to "heck yeah!"

Chapter 1: The Pegan Diet Philosophy

In the realm of nutrition, the Pegan Diet emerges as a distinctive and effective approach to healthy eating. Blending the best aspects of both paleo and vegan dietary patterns, the Pegan Diet advocates an abundance of whole, plant-based foods while incorporating moderate amounts of animal protein. This balanced approach offers a plethora of health advantages, including weight management, improved gut health, and reduced risk of chronic diseases.

Origins and Evolution

The Pegan Diet concept was introduced by Dr. Mark Hyman, a renowned functional medicine physician, in his book "The Pegan Diet: Food for Health and Longevity." Dr. Hyman recognized the potential benefits of combining elements from both paleo and vegan diets, aiming to create a dietary pattern that could address the nutritional needs of individuals seeking optimal health.

Core Principles

The Pegan Diet is founded on several key principles that guide its overall philosophy:

1. **Emphasis on Whole Foods**: The diet emphasizes the consumption of whole, unprocessed foods that align with the natural diet of our ancestors. Fruits, vegetables, nuts, seeds, and legumes fall under this category.

2. **Moderate Animal Protein**: While primarily plant-based, the Pegan Diet allows for moderate intake of animal protein from high-quality sources. This includes grass-fed meats, pasture-raised eggs, and wild-caught fish.

3. **Elimination of Processed Foods**: Highly processed foods, refined grains, artificial sweeteners, and excessive amounts of added sugar are discouraged due to their potential negative impact on health.

4. **Focus on Nutrient Density**: The Pegan Diet prioritizes nutrient-dense foods that provide a rich supply of vitamins, minerals, fiber, and antioxidants.

5. Mindful Eating: The diet encourages mindful eating practices, promoting awareness of hunger cues and savoring each bite.

Benefits of the Pegan Diet

Numerous possible health benefits of the Pegan diet include:

1. **Weight Management**: The diet's emphasis on whole, fiber-rich foods and moderate protein intake can support healthy weight management.
2. **Improved Gut Health**: The abundance of plant-based foods promotes a healthy gut microbiome, which plays a crucial role in overall health.
3. **Reduced Risk of Chronic Diseases**: The Pegan Diet's nutrient-dense foods and balanced approach may help lower the risk of chronic diseases such as heart disease, diabetes, and certain types of cancer.
4. **Enhanced Energy Levels**: The diet's focus on whole, unprocessed foods can contribute to sustained energy levels throughout the day.
5. **Improved Mood and Cognitive Function**: The nutritional profile of the Pegan Diet

may support positive mood and cognitive function.

Navigating the Pegan Diet

Adopting the Pegan Diet may involve some initial adjustments, but with planning and commitment, it can become a sustainable and enjoyable way of eating. Here are some tips for successfully navigating the Pegan Diet:

1. **Make Gradual Changes**: Gradually introduce Pegan principles into your diet, allowing your body to adapt to the new food patterns.
2. **Seek Guidance**: Consult a healthcare professional or registered dietitian for personalized advice and support.
3. **Explore Recipes**: Utilize Pegan recipes and cookbooks to discover delicious and nutritious meal options.
4. **Embrace Variety**: Incorporate a wide range of fruits, vegetables, nuts, seeds, and legumes to ensure a balanced and nutrient-rich diet.
5. **Cook at Home**: Cooking more meals at home allows you to control ingredients and ensure adherence to Pegan principles.

6. **Practice mindful eating: Notice when you're hungry, enjoy every mouthful, and keep your eyes off other things while you eat.**
7. **Plan Ahead**: Plan your meals and snacks for the week to avoid unhealthy choices when hunger strikes.
8. **Be Patient**: It takes time to develop new habits and fully integrate the Pegan Diet into your lifestyle.

By embracing the Pegan Diet philosophy and incorporating its principles into your daily life, you can embark on a journey towards enhanced health, vitality, and overall well-being.

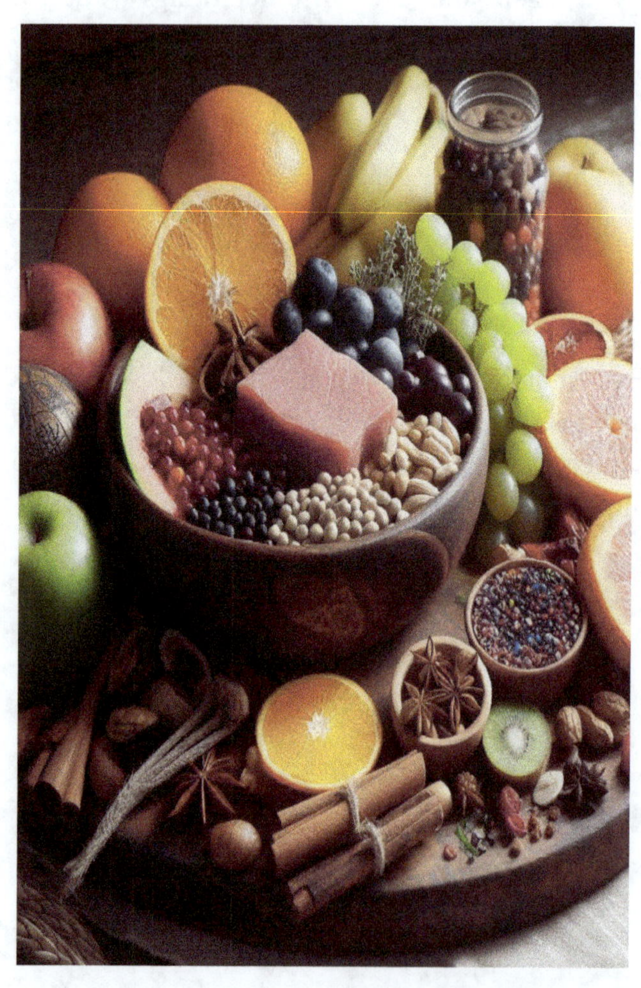

Chapter 2: Pegan Diet Essentials

The Pegan Diet encompasses a diverse array of nutrient-rich foods that nourish the body and promote optimal health. By understanding the essential components of this dietary pattern, you can make informed choices and reap the full benefits of the Pegan lifestyle.

Fruits and Vegetables: The Foundation of the Pegan Diet

Fruits and vegetables form the cornerstone of the Pegan Diet, providing a wealth of essential vitamins, minerals, and fiber. These nutrient-dense powerhouses play a crucial role in maintaining overall health and reducing the risk of chronic diseases.

- **Fruits**: Aim for a variety of colorful fruits, including berries, citrus fruits, apples, pears, and bananas. These fruits provide a rich source of antioxidants, vitamins C and E, and potassium, all of which contribute to overall well-being.

- **Vegetables**: Fill your plate with a vibrant array of vegetables, including leafy greens, cruciferous vegetables (broccoli, cauliflower, kale), root vegetables (carrots, beets, sweet potatoes), and nightshades (tomatoes, peppers, eggplant). These vegetables offer an abundance of vitamins A, K, and folate, along with fiber and essential minerals.

Nuts and Seeds: Nature's Tiny Powerhouses

Nuts and seeds are nutritional superstars, packed with healthy fats, protein, fiber, and antioxidants. These nutrient-dense snacks provide sustained energy, promote satiety, and support heart health.

- **Nuts**: Incorporate a variety of nuts into your diet, such as almonds, walnuts, pecans, pistachios, and macadamia nuts. These nuts offer a rich source of omega-3 fatty acids, vitamin E, and magnesium.

- **Seeds**: Sprinkle seeds like chia seeds, flaxseeds, pumpkin seeds, and sunflower seeds into your snacks, salads, and smoothies. These seeds provide a wealth of fiber, healthy fats, and essential minerals.

Legumes: Plant-Based Protein Powerhouses

Legumes, including beans, lentils, and peas, are excellent sources of plant-based protein, fiber, and complex carbohydrates. These versatile ingredients can be incorporated into soups, stews, salads, and main dishes.

- **Beans**: Explore a variety of beans, such as kidney beans, black beans, pinto beans, and chickpeas. These beans provide a rich source of protein, fiber, iron, and B vitamins.

- **Lentils**: Consider lentils as a staple in your Pegan Diet. Red lentils, green lentils, and brown lentils offer a high concentration of protein, fiber, and essential nutrients.

- **Peas**: Include peas in your diet, such as green peas, split peas, and snow peas. These peas offer a combination of protein, fiber, vitamins A and C, and potassium.

Grass-Fed Meats, Pasture-Raised Eggs, and Wild-Caught Fish: Animal Protein Sources

While the Pegan Diet emphasizes plant-based foods, it also allows for moderate intake of animal protein from high-quality sources. These options provide essential amino acids and other nutrients that support overall health.

- **Grass-Fed Meats**: Choose grass-fed meats, such as beef, bison, and lamb, for their superior nutrient profile. Grass-fed meats are higher in omega-3 fatty acids, conjugated linoleic acid (CLA), and antioxidants compared to grain-fed meats.

- **Pasture-Raised Eggs**: Opt for pasture-raised eggs, which are richer in omega-3 fatty acids, vitamin D, and other nutrients compared to conventionally raised eggs.

- **Wild-Caught Fish**: Select wild-caught fish, such as salmon, tuna, sardines, and mackerel, for their high concentration of omega-3 fatty acids, protein, and vitamin D.

Balancing Macronutrients

The Pegan Diet aims to achieve a balanced macronutrient profile, promoting a healthy relationship with food and preventing nutritional deficiencies.

- **Carbohydrates**: Prioritize complex carbohydrates from whole grains, fruits, vegetables, and legumes. These carbs supply necessary minerals and long-lasting energy.

- **Protein**: Include moderate amounts of protein from plant and animal sources. Protein supports muscle growth, tissue repair, and various bodily functions.

- **Fats**: Emphasize healthy fats from nuts, seeds, avocados, and olive oil. These fats contribute to heart health, brain function, and nutrient absorption.

- **Fiber**: Aim for a high intake of fiber from fruits, vegetables, legumes, and whole grains. Fiber promotes digestive health, blood sugar control, and satiety.

By incorporating these essential foods and balancing macronutrients, you can create a Pegan Diet that aligns with your individual needs and preferences.

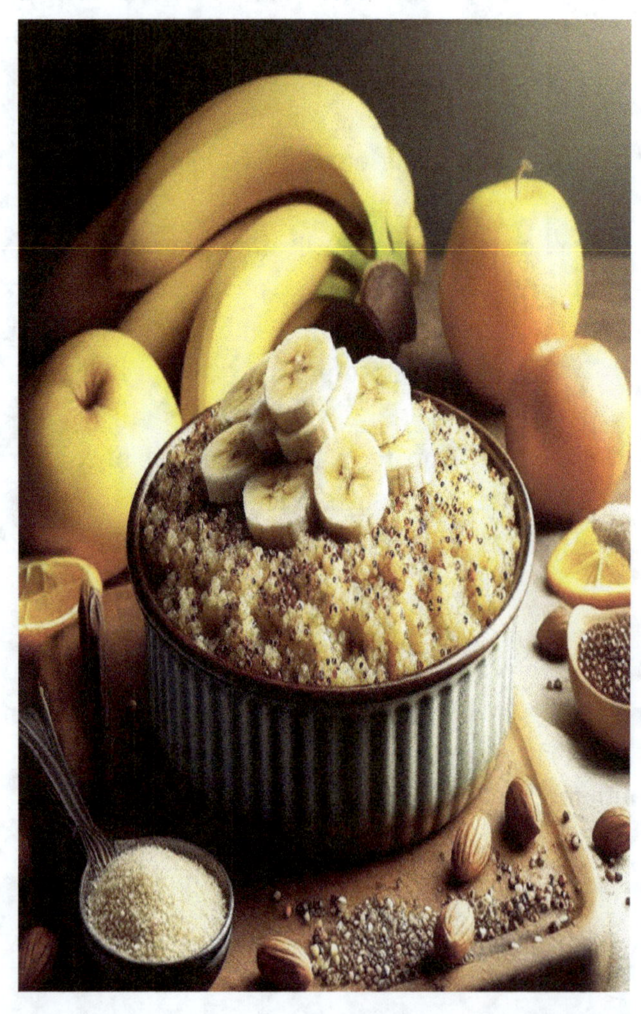

Chapter 3: Breakfast

Banana-Infused Quinoa Bake

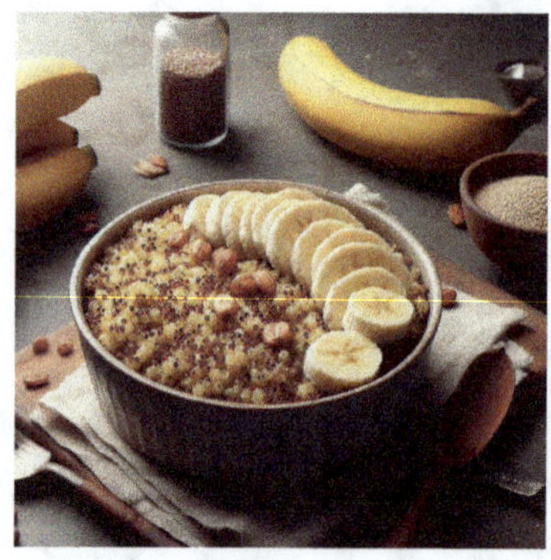

Preparation Time: 10 minutes
Cooking Time: 30 minutes
Servings: 4

Ingredients:
- 1 cup quinoa
- 2 cups water
- 2 ripe bananas, mashed
- 1/4 cup almond milk
- 1 teaspoon cinnamon
- 1/4 teaspoon nutmeg
- 1 tablespoon of maple syrup or honey, (if desired)
- Sliced bananas and nuts for topping (optional)

Directions:
1. Preheat oven to 350°F (175°C).

2. Rinse quinoa and combine with water in a saucepan. After bringing to a boil, lower the heat, and simmer, covered, for fifteen minutes.

3. In a bowl, mix cooked quinoa, mashed bananas, almond milk, cinnamon, nutmeg, and sweetener (if using).

4. Transfer mixture to a baking dish. If desired, garnish with chopped nuts and bananas.

5. Bake until it starts to turn brown, (this should take about 15 to 20 minutes).

6. Serve warm and enjoy!

Nutritional Value (per serving):
Calories: 220 | Carbs: 44g |
Protein: 6g | Fat: 3g | Fiber: 5g

Chia Berry Overnight Oats

Prep Time: 5 minutes | Cooking Time: No cooking required | Servings: 2

Ingredients:
- 1 cup rolled oats
- 2 tablespoons chia seeds
- 1 1/2 cups almond milk (or any preferred milk)
- 1 cup mixed berries (strawberries, blueberries, raspberries)
- 1 tablespoon of maple syrup or honey, (if desired)
- Nuts or seeds for topping (optional)

Directions:
1. In a jar or bowl, combine rolled oats, chia seeds, almond milk, and sweetener (if using). Stir well.
2. Add mixed berries to the mixture and gently mix them in.
3. Cover and refrigerate overnight or for at least 4 hours.
4. Before serving, stir well and add toppings like nuts or seeds if desired.

Nutritional Value (per serving):
Calories: 280 | Carbs: 46g |
Protein: 8g | Fat: 7g | Fiber: 10g

Hearty Barley Porridge

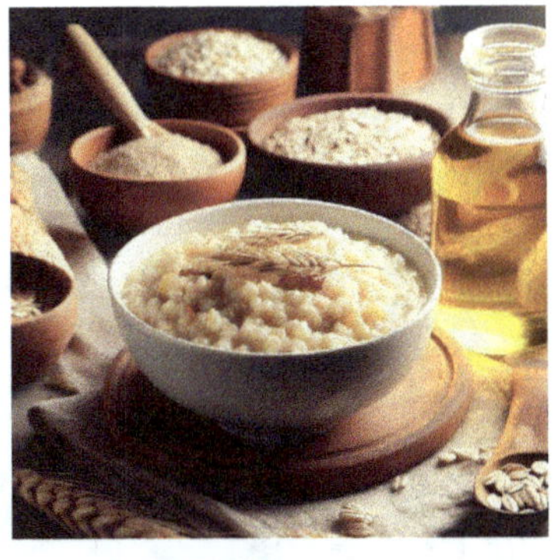

Preparation Time: 5 minutes
Cooking Time: 40 minutes
Servings: 4

Ingredients:
- 1 cup pearl barley
- 3 cups water
- 2 glasses almond milk (or your favorite kind)
- 1 teaspoon vanilla extract
- 1/4 teaspoon cinnamon
- 2 tablespoon of maple syrup or honey, (if desired)
- Sliced fruits or nuts for topping (optional)

Directions:
1. Run some water over the pearl barley to rinse it.
2. Put the barley and water in a saucepan. After bringing to a boil, lower the heat to a simmer. Cook for 30-40 minutes or until the barley is tender and most of the liquid is absorbed.

3. Stir in almond milk, vanilla extract, cinnamon, and sweetener (if using). Cook for an additional 5-10 minutes, stirring occasionally, until the mixture thickens.

4. Take off from the heat and allow to cool a bit.

5. Serve warm, topped with sliced fruits or nuts if desired.

Nutritional Value (per serving):
Calories: 240 | Carbs: 50g |
Protein: 6g | Fat: 3g | Fiber: 8g

Scrambled Breakfast Tacos

Preparation Time: 10 minutes
Cooking Time: 15 minutes
Servings: 4

Ingredients:
- 8 large eggs
- 1 tablespoon olive oil
- 1 bell pepper, diced
- 1 small onion, diced
- 1 cup cherry tomatoes, halved
- 1 teaspoon chili powder
- Salt and pepper to taste
- 1/2 cup shredded cheddar cheese
- 4 whole wheat tortillas
- Avocado slices, salsa, or cilantro for topping (optional)

Directions:
1. Whisk the eggs in a dish and set it aside.
2. In a pan over medium heat, warm the olive oil. Add onion and bell pepper, and cook until softened.
3. Add cherry tomatoes, chili powder, salt, and pepper. Cook for a few minutes.

4. Pour in the whisked eggs and cook, stirring occasionally until eggs are scrambled and cooked through.

5. Sprinkle shredded cheese on top and let it melt.

6. Serve the scramble in whole wheat tortillas. Add optional toppings like avocado, salsa, or cilantro if desired.

Nutritional Value (per serving):
Calories: 300 | Carbs: 18g |
Protein: 18g | Fat: 18g | Fiber: 4g

Wholesome Feta Egg Bake

Preparation Time: 10 minutes
Cooking Time: 20 minutes
Servings: 6

Ingredients:
- 8 large eggs
- 1/4 cup milk
- 1 cup spinach, chopped
- 1/2 cup cherry tomatoes, halved
- 1/2 cup crumbled feta cheese
- Salt and pepper to taste
- 1 tablespoon olive oil

Directions:
1. Preheat oven to 350°F (175°C).
2. In a bowl, whisk together eggs, milk, salt, and pepper.
3. Heat olive oil in an oven-safe skillet over medium heat.
4. Add spinach and cherry tomatoes, sauté until spinach wilts.
5. Transfer the beaten eggs into the skillet. Cook until the edges begin to set, (this should take only a few minutes).

6. Sprinkle feta cheese evenly over the top.
7. Transfer the skillet to the oven and bake for 12-15 minutes until the frittata is set.
8. Slice and serve.

Nutritional Value (per serving):
Calories: 160 | Carbs: 3g |
Protein: 11g | Fat: 11g | Fiber: 1g

Mixed Farro Salad

Preparation Time: 15 minutes
Cooking Time: 25 minutes (for farro)
Servings: 4

Ingredients:
- 1 cup farro
- 2½ cups veggie broth or water
- 1 cucumber, diced
- 1 cup cherry tomatoes, halved
- 1/4 cup red onion, finely chopped
- 1/4 cup fresh parsley, chopped
- 1/4 cup feta cheese, crumbled
- 2 tablespoons olive oil
- 2 tablespoons lemon juice
- Salt and pepper to taste

Directions:
1. Rinse farro under running water. Bring broth or water to a boil in a saucepan. Add farro, reduce heat, cover, and simmer for 20-25 minutes until tender. Drain excess liquid if needed.
2. In a large bowl, combine cooked farro, cucumber, cherry tomatoes, red onion, parsley, and feta cheese.

3. Mix the olive oil, lemon juice, salt, and pepper in a different small bowl.

4. Drizzle the salad with the dressing and mix thoroughly.

5. Serve chilled or at room temperature.

Nutritional Value (per serving):
Calories: 280 | Carbs: 38g
Protein: 8g | Fat: 11g | Fiber: 6g

Italian Style Veggie Salad

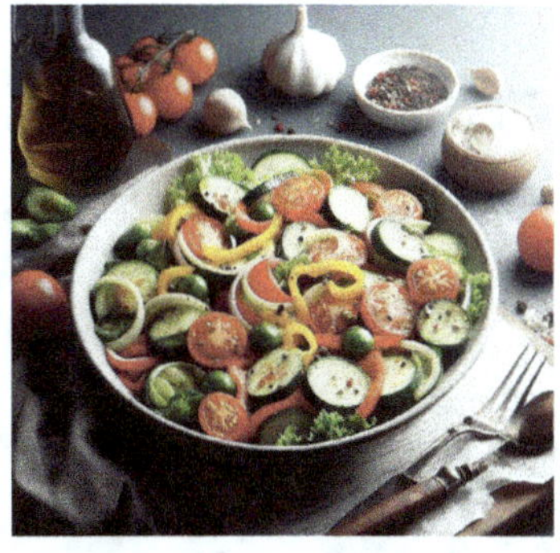

Preparation Time: 15 minutes
Cooking Time: No cooking required
Servings: 4

Ingredients:
- 2 cups mixed salad greens
- 1 cup cherry tomatoes, halved
- 1/2 cup cucumber, sliced
- 1/4 cup red onion, thinly sliced
- 1/4 cup black olives, sliced
- 1/4 cup feta cheese, crumbled
- 2 tablespoons olive oil
- 2 tablespoons balsamic vinegar
- 1 teaspoon dried oregano
- Salt and pepper to taste

Directions:

1. In a large bowl, combine mixed salad greens, cherry tomatoes, cucumber, red onion, black olives, and feta cheese.

2. In a small bowl, whisk together olive oil, balsamic vinegar, dried oregano, salt, and pepper.

3. Drizzle the salad with the dressing and mix gently to coat.

4. Serve immediately as a refreshing side or main dish.

Nutritional Value (per serving):
Calories: 150 | Carbs: 8g |
Protein: 4g | Fat: 12g | Fiber: 2g

Creamy Spinach Tofu Salad

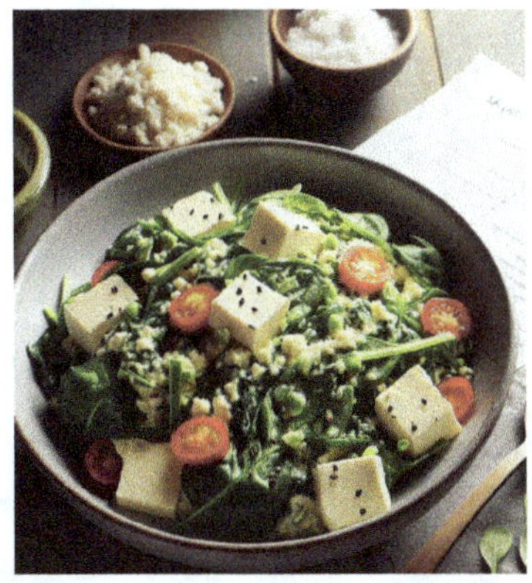

Preparation Time: 15 minutes
Cooking Time: No cooking required
Servings: 2

Ingredients:
- 2 cups fresh spinach leaves
- 1/2 cup firm tofu, mashed
- 1/4 cup cherry tomatoes, halved
- 1/4 cup cucumber, diced
- 2 tablespoons red onion, finely chopped
- 2 tablespoons sunflower seeds
- 2 tablespoons olive oil
- 1 tablespoon balsamic vinegar
- Salt and pepper to taste

Directions:

1. In a bowl, combine fresh spinach, mashed tofu, cherry tomatoes, cucumber, red onion, and sunflower seeds.

2. In a separate small bowl, whisk together olive oil, balsamic vinegar, salt, and pepper.

3. Drizzle the dressing over the salad and toss gently to combine.

4. Serve immediately as a nutritious salad.

Nutritional Value (per serving):
Calories: 200 | Carbs: 8g |
Protein: 10g | Fat: 15g | Fiber: 3g

Crispy Muesli Delight

Preparation Time: 10 minutes
Cooking Time: No cooking required
Servings: 4

Ingredients:
- 2 cups rolled oats
- 1/2 cup almonds, chopped
- 1/4 cup sunflower seeds
- 1/4 cup pumpkin seeds
- 1/4 cup dried cranberries or raisins
- 1/4 cup honey or maple syrup
- 1 teaspoon vanilla extract
- 1/2 teaspoon cinnamon
- 1/4 teaspoon salt

Directions:
1. In a large mixing bowl, combine rolled oats, almonds, sunflower seeds, pumpkin seeds, and dried cranberries or raisins.
2. In a separate small bowl, mix together honey or maple syrup, vanilla extract, cinnamon, and salt.
3. Pour the liquid mixture over the dry ingredients and stir until well coated.

4. Spread the mixture evenly on a baking sheet and bake at 300°F (150°C) for 25-30 minutes, stirring halfway through.

5. Let it cool completely and store in an airtight container.

Nutritional Value (per serving):
Calories: 300 | Carbs: 40g |
Protein: 8g | Fat: 13g | Fiber: 6g

Bacon Veggie Omelet

Preparation Time: 10 minutes
Cooking Time: 10 minutes
Servings: 2

Ingredients:
- 4 large eggs
- 4 slices bacon, chopped
- 1/2 cup bell peppers, diced
- 1/4 cup onion, finely chopped
- 1/2 cup spinach, chopped
- Salt and pepper to taste
- 2 tablespoons shredded cheese (optional)

Directions:
1. In a bowl, beat the eggs. Season with salt and pepper.
2. Crisp up bacon by cooking it in a skillet over medium heat. If necessary, remove extra grease.
3. Add onion and bell peppers to skillet. Cook until the food becomes tender.
4. Add chopped spinach to the skillet and cook until wilted.
5. Pour beaten eggs evenly over the veggies and bacon. Cook until the edges start to set.

6. If using, sprinkle shredded cheese over one half of the omelet.

7. Gently fold the omelet in half and cook for another minute until cheese melts and eggs are fully cooked.

8. Serve hot and enjoy!

Nutritional Value (per serving):
Calories: 320 | Carbs: 4g |
Protein: 18g | Fat: 25g | Fiber: 1g

Chapter 4: Lunch

Baked Acorn Squash Delight

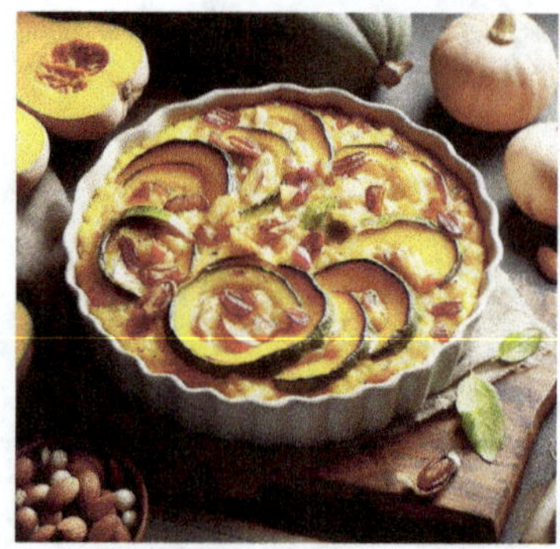

Preparation Time: 20 minutes
Cooking Time: 1 hour
Servings: 6

Ingredients:
- 2 acorn squashes, halved and seeded
- 1 tablespoon olive oil
- 1 onion, diced
- 2 cloves garlic, minced
- 1 bell pepper, diced
- 1 cup cooked quinoa
- 1 cup cooked black beans
- 1 teaspoon cumin
- 1 teaspoon paprika
- Salt and pepper to taste
- 1/2 cup shredded cheese (optional)
- Chopped cilantro for garnish (optional)

Directions:

1. Preheat oven to 375°F (190°C).

2. Place acorn squash halves on a baking sheet, cut side down. Bake squash for 30 to 40 minutes, or until soft.

3. In a pan over medium heat, warm the olive oil. Add onion, garlic, and bell pepper. Sauté until softened.

4. Stir in cooked quinoa, black beans, cumin, paprika, salt, and pepper.

5. Scoop the quinoa mixture into the cooked acorn squash halves.

6. Sprinkle shredded cheese on top if desired and return to the oven for 10-15 minutes until heated through.

7. Garnish with chopped cilantro before serving.

Nutritional Value (per serving):
Calories: 230 | Carbs: 40g |
Protein: 8g | Fat: 5g | Fiber: 8g

Spicy Cajun Collard Greens

Preparation Time: 15 minutes
Cooking Time: 45 minutes
Servings: 4

Ingredients:
- 1 bunch collard greens, stems removed and leaves chopped
- 4 slices bacon, chopped
- 1 onion, diced
- 2 cloves garlic, minced
- 1 teaspoon Cajun seasoning
- 1/2 teaspoon smoked paprika
- Salt and pepper to taste
- 1 cup chicken or vegetable broth

Directions:
1. Cook bacon in a Dutch oven or big saucepan over medium heat until crispy. While leaving the bacon grease in the saucepan, remove the bacon and set it aside.
2. Add chopped onion to saucepan and cook till it becomes transparent. Cook for one more minute after adding the minced garlic.

3. Stir in chopped collard greens, Cajun seasoning, smoked paprika, salt, and pepper. Cook for 5 minutes, stirring occasionally.

4. Pour in chicken or vegetable broth, cover, and simmer for 30-40 minutes until collard greens are tender.

5. Stir in the cooked bacon before serving.

Nutritional Value (per serving):
Calories: 120 | Carbs: 10g |
Protein: 6g | Fat: 7g | Fiber: 4g

Beef Infusion with Broccoli

Preparation Time: 15 minutes
Cooking Time: 20 minutes
Servings: 4

Ingredients:
- 1 pound flank steak, sliced thinly
- 3 cups broccoli florets
- 2 tablespoons soy sauce
- 2 tablespoons oyster sauce
- 2 cloves garlic, minced
- 1 teaspoon ginger, grated
- 1 tablespoon cornstarch
- 2 tablespoons oil for stir-frying

Directions:
1. In a bowl, mix soy sauce, oyster sauce, minced garlic, grated ginger, and cornstarch. Marinate the sliced beef in this mixture for 10-15 minutes.
2. In a skillet or wok, heat the oil over high heat. Add marinated beef and stir-fry for 2-3 minutes until browned. Remove beef from the skillet.
3. In the same skillet, add broccoli florets and stir-fry for 3-4 minutes until tender-crisp.

4. Return the beef to the skillet and stir-fry for another minute until everything is heated through.
5. Serve hot with rice or noodles.

Nutritional Value (per serving):
Calories: 280 | Carbs: 9g |
Protein: 25g | Fat: 15g | Fiber: 3g

Salmon Delight Omelet

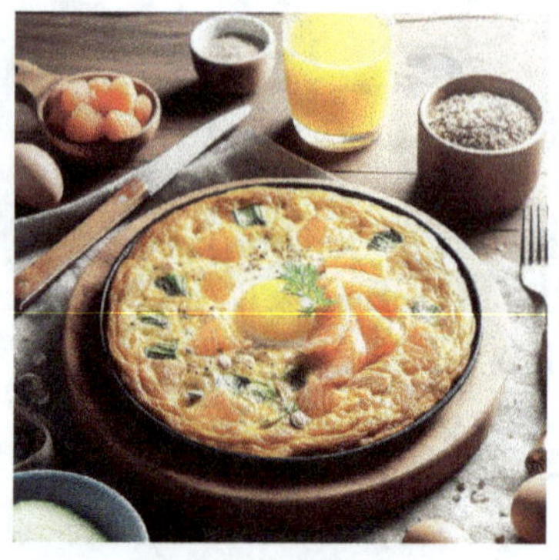

Preparation Time: 10 minutes
Cooking Time: 10 minutes
Servings: 2

Ingredients:
- 4 large eggs
- 1/2 cup cooked salmon, flaked
- 1/4 cup red bell pepper, diced
- 2 tablespoons red onion, finely chopped
- 2 tablespoons cream cheese
- Salt and pepper to taste
- 1 tablespoon butter or oil for cooking

Directions:

1. In a bowl, beat the eggs. Add flaked salmon, diced red bell pepper, red onion, cream cheese, salt, and pepper. Mix well.

2. In a skillet, heat the oil or butter over medium heat. Transfer the egg mixture in.

3. Cook for 2-3 minutes until the edges start to set. Gently lift the edges and tilt the skillet to let the uncooked egg flow underneath.

4. When the omelet is mostly set but still slightly runny in the center, fold it in half.

5. Cook for another minute until the center sets.

6. Transfer the omelet to a plate and serve.

Nutritional Value (per serving):
Calories: 320 | Carbs: 4g |
Protein: 25g | Fat: 22g | Fiber: 1g

Flavorful Curry Chicken Salad

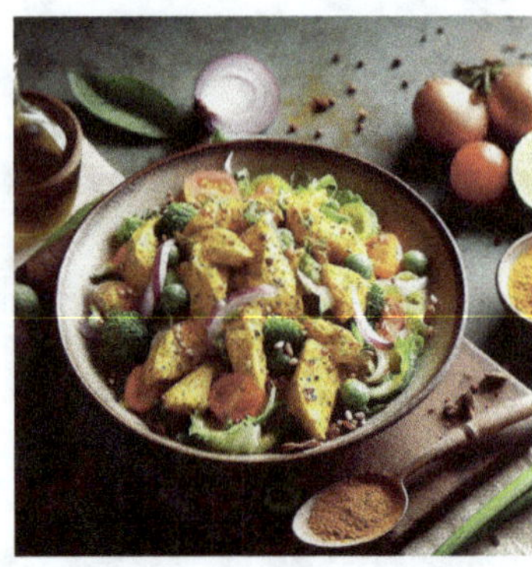

Preparation Time: 15 minutes
Cooking Time: 20 minutes (for chicken)
Servings: 4

Ingredients:
- 2 chicken breasts, cooked and shredded
- 1/2 cup Greek yogurt
- 2 tablespoons mayonnaise
- 1 tablespoon curry powder
- 1/4 cup red onion, finely chopped
- 1/4 cup celery, diced
- 1/4 cup grapes, halved
- Salt and pepper to taste
- Lettuce leaves for serving (optional)

Directions:
1. In a bowl, mix shredded chicken, Greek yogurt, mayonnaise, curry powder, red onion, celery, grapes, salt, and pepper until well combined.

2. Refrigerate for at least 30 minutes to let the flavors meld.

3. Serve on lettuce leaves as a salad or use it as a sandwich filling.

Nutritional Value (per serving):
Calories: 230 | Carbs: 6g |
Protein: 25g | Fat: 10g | Fiber: 1g

Savory Swedish Meatballs

Preparation Time: 20 minutes
Cooking Time: 20 minutes
Servings: 4

Ingredients:
- 1 pound ground beef
- 1/2 cup breadcrumbs
- 1/4 cup milk
- 1 egg
- 1/4 cup onion, finely chopped
- 1 clove garlic, minced
- 1/2 teaspoon salt
- 1/4 teaspoon black pepper
- 1/4 teaspoon nutmeg
- 2 tablespoons butter
- 2 tablespoons flour
- 1 cup beef broth
- 1/2 cup heavy cream
- 1 tablespoon Worcestershire sauce
- Chopped parsley for garnish (optional)

Directions:
1. In a bowl, combine ground beef, breadcrumbs, milk, egg, chopped onion, minced garlic, salt,

pepper, and nutmeg. Combine well and shape into meatballs.

2. Over medium heat, melt butter in a pan. Add meatballs and cook until browned on all sides and cooked through, for about 10-12 minutes. Remove meatballs from the skillet and set aside.

3. In the same skillet, add flour and stir for 1-2 minutes until golden brown.

4. Slowly pour in beef broth while stirring continuously to avoid lumps. Add heavy cream and Worcestershire sauce. Simmer until the sauce thickens.

5. Return the meatballs to the skillet and simmer for another 5 minutes in the sauce.

6. Garnish with chopped parsley before serving.

Nutritional Value (per serving):
Calories: 380 | Carbs: 12g |
Protein: 22g | Fat: 26g | Fiber: 1g

Avocado Infused Shrimp Salad

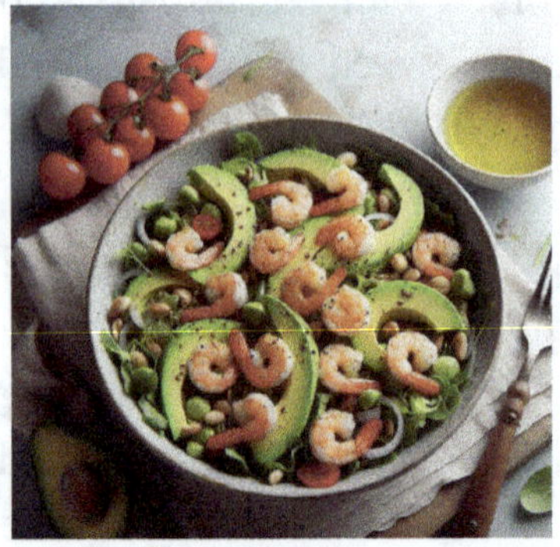

Preparation Time: 15 minutes
Cooking Time: 5 minutes (for shrimp)
Servings: 2

Ingredients:
- 10-12 large shrimp, peeled and deveined
- 2 avocados, diced
- 1 cup cherry tomatoes, halved
- 1/4 cup red onion, finely chopped
- 1/4 cup cilantro, chopped
- 2 tablespoons lime juice
- 2 tablespoons olive oil
- Salt and pepper to taste

Directions:

1. Season shrimp with salt and pepper. Heat olive oil in a skillet over medium-high heat. Cook shrimp for 2-3 minutes per side until pink and cooked through. Remove from heat and set aside.

2. In a bowl, combine diced avocados, cherry tomatoes, red onion, and chopped cilantro.
3. Add cooked shrimp to the bowl.
4. Drizzle lime juice and olive oil over the salad. Gently toss to combine.
5. Serve immediately as a refreshing salad.

Nutritional Value (per serving):
Calories: 350 | Carbs: 18g |
Protein: 16g | Fat: 26g | Fiber: 12g

Chicken Lettuce Wraps

Preparation Time: 15 minutes
Cooking Time: 15 minutes
Servings: 4

Ingredients:
- 1 pound ground chicken
- 2 tablespoons oil
- 1 onion, diced
- 2 cloves garlic, minced
- 1 bell pepper, diced
- 1/4 cup hoisin sauce
- 2 tablespoons soy sauce
- 1 tablespoon rice vinegar
- 1 teaspoon sesame oil
- 1 can water chestnuts, drained and chopped
- 1 head iceberg or butter lettuce, leaves separated

Directions:
1. In a skillet, heat the oil over medium-high heat. Add ground chicken and cook until browned.
2. Add diced onion, minced garlic, and diced bell pepper. Sauté for a few minutes until vegetables are tender.

3. Stir in hoisin sauce, soy sauce, rice vinegar, sesame oil, and chopped water chestnuts. Cook for another 2-3 minutes until heated through.

4. Spoon the chicken mixture onto lettuce leaves, creating wraps.

5. Serve immediately and enjoy the flavorful wraps.

Nutritional Value (per serving):
Calories: 280 | Carbs: 14g |
Protein: 20g | Fat: 16g | Fiber: 4g

Savory Pork Rice Strips

Preparation Time: 15 minutes
Cooking Time: 25 minutes
Servings: 4

Ingredients:
- 1 pound pork loin, cut into strips
- 2 cups cooked rice
- 1 onion, sliced
- 2 cloves garlic, minced
- 1 bell pepper, sliced
- 2 tablespoons soy sauce
- 1 tablespoon oyster sauce
- 1 tablespoon vegetable oil
- Salt and pepper to taste
- Chopped green onions for garnish (optional)

Directions:
1. Heat vegetable oil in a skillet or wok over medium-high heat. Add pork strips and cook until browned on all sides. Remove pork from the skillet and set aside.
2. In the same skillet, sauté sliced onion and minced garlic until softened.

3. Add sliced bell pepper to the skillet and stir-fry for a few minutes.

4. Return the pork to the skillet. Add soy sauce and oyster sauce. Stir-fry for a further two to three minutes, or until well heated.

5. Top cooked rice with pork slices. If desired, add some chopped green onions as a garnish.

Nutritional Value (per serving):
Calories: 380 | Carbs: 30g |
Protein: 25g | Fat: 15g | Fiber: 2g

Mediterranean Seasoned Lamb Chops

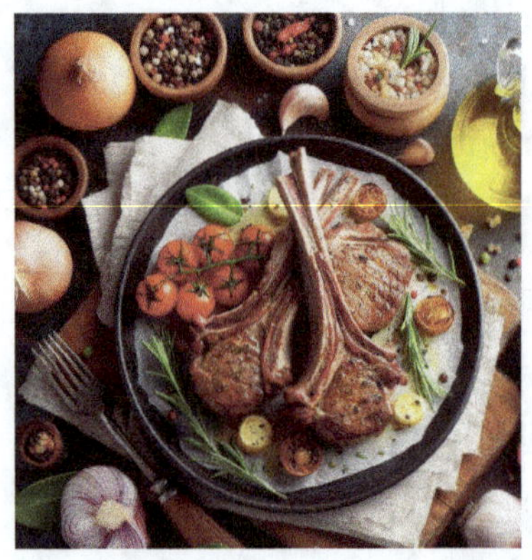

Preparation Time: 10 minutes
Cooking Time: 10 minutes
Servings: 2

Ingredients:
- 4 lamb chops
- 2 tablespoons olive oil
- 2 cloves garlic, minced
- 1 teaspoon dried oregano
- 1 teaspoon dried thyme
- Salt and pepper to taste
- Lemon wedges for garnish

Directions:
1. Preheat grill or skillet over medium-high heat.
2. In a bowl, mix olive oil, minced garlic, dried oregano, dried thyme, salt, and pepper.

3. Rub the mixture onto both sides of the lamb chops.

4. Grill or pan-sear lamb chops for about 4-5 minutes per side for medium-rare or until desired doneness.

5. Let the chops rest for a few minutes before serving.

6. Garnish with lemon wedges and enjoy!

Nutritional Value (per serving):
Calories: 350 | Carbs: 1g |
Protein: 25g | Fat: 28g | Fiber: 0g

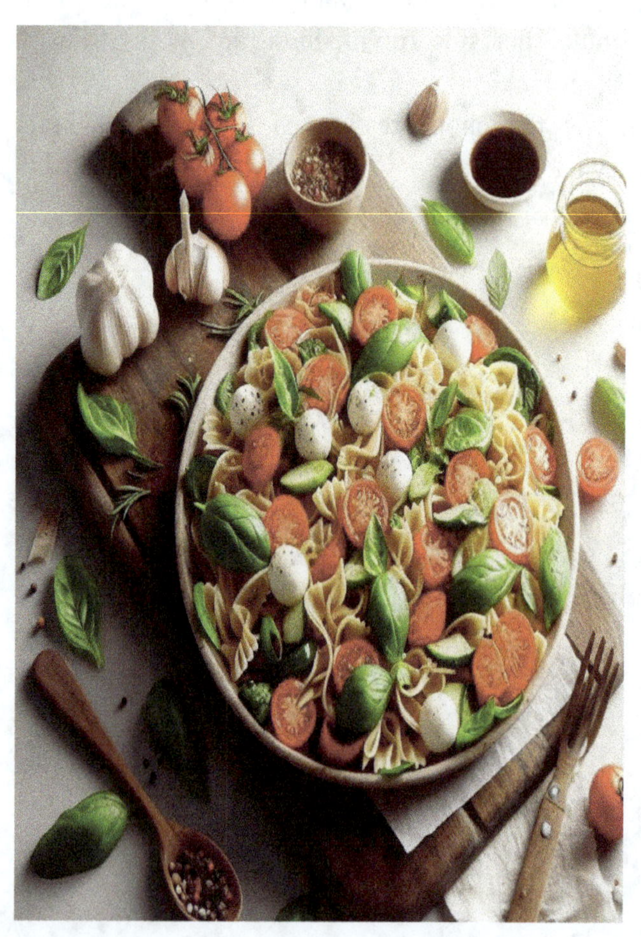

Chapter 5: Dinner

Creamy White Bean Soup

Preparation Time: 10 minutes
Cooking Time: 30 minutes
Servings: 6

Ingredients:
- 2 washed and drained cans of white beans
- 1 onion, chopped
- 2 cloves garlic, minced
- 2 carrots, diced
- 2 celery stalks, diced
- 4 cups vegetable or chicken broth
- 1 teaspoon dried thyme
- 1 teaspoon dried rosemary
- Salt and pepper to taste
- Olive oil for sautéing
- Chopped parsley for garnish (optional)

Directions:
1. In a saucepan over medium heat, warm the olive oil. When fragrant, add the chopped onion and garlic and sauté.
2. Add celery and chopped carrots. Cook for a few minutes until they begin to soften.
3. Add the broth and heat until it simmers.

4. Add white beans, dried thyme, dried rosemary, salt, and pepper. Simmer for 20-25 minutes.

5. Use an immersion blender or transfer a portion of the soup to a blender and blend until smooth (optional for a creamier consistency).

6. Serve hot, garnished with chopped parsley if desired.

Nutritional Value (per serving):
Calories: 200 | Carbs: 35g |
Protein: 10g | Fat: 2g | Fiber: 10g

Juicy Lamb Burgers

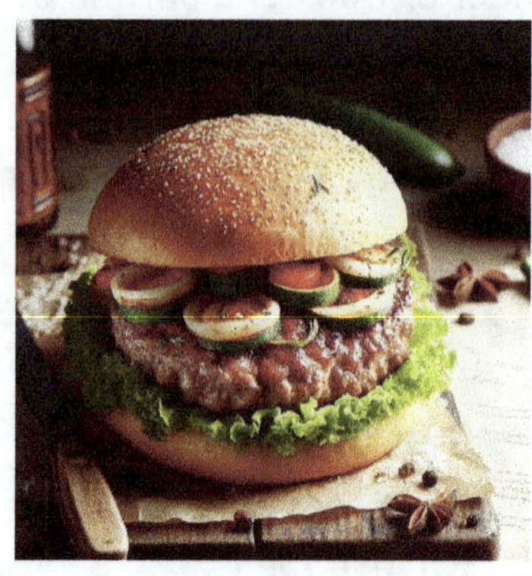

Preparation Time: 15 minutes
Cooking Time: 10 minutes
Servings: 4

Ingredients:
- 1 pound ground lamb
- 4 burger buns
- 1 tomato, sliced
- 1 red onion, sliced
- Lettuce leaves
- 4 tablespoons tzatziki sauce
- Salt and pepper to taste

Directions:
1. Divide ground lamb into four equal portions and shape them into patties.
2. Season each patty with salt and pepper.

3. Heat a grill or skillet over medium-high heat. Cook the lamb patties for about 4-5 minutes per side or until desired doneness.

4. Toast burger buns lightly on the grill or in a toaster.

5. Assemble the burgers: place lettuce leaves on the bottom bun, followed by the lamb patty, tomato slices, red onion slices, and a dollop of tzatziki sauce. Top with the other half of the bun.

6. Serve hot and enjoy!

Nutritional Value (per serving):
Calories: 450 | Carbs: 25g |
Protein: 25g | Fat: 25g | Fiber: 3g

Quinoa Chicken Fusion Bowls

Preparation Time: 15 minutes
Cooking Time: 25 minutes
Servings: 4

Ingredients:
- 1 cup quinoa
- 2 cups chicken broth
- 1 pound chicken breasts, sliced
- 2 tablespoons olive oil
- 1 teaspoon paprika
- 1 teaspoon garlic powder
- Salt and pepper to taste
- 2 cups mixed vegetables (bell peppers, broccoli, etc.)
- Avocado slices for topping
- Lemon wedges for garnish

Directions:
1. Rinse quinoa and cook in chicken broth according to package instructions.
2. Season chicken slices with paprika, garlic powder, salt, and pepper.
3. Heat olive oil in a skillet over medium-high heat. Cook the chicken until browned and cooked

through, about 5-6 minutes per side. Take out of the skillet and place it aside.

4. In the same skillet, sauté mixed vegetables until tender-crisp.

5. Assemble bowls: divide cooked quinoa among bowls, top with cooked chicken slices, sautéed vegetables, and avocado slices.

6. Garnish with lemon wedges and serve.

Nutritional Value (per serving):
Calories: 380 | Carbs: 30g |
Protein: 30g | Fat: 15g | Fiber: 6g

Citrusy Cilantro Shrimp

Prep Time: 10 minutes | Cooking Time: 5 minutes | Servings: 2

Ingredients:
- 12-16 large shrimp, peeled and deveined
- Zest and juice of 1 lemon
- 2 cloves garlic, minced
- 1/4 cup chopped cilantro
- 2 tablespoons olive oil
- Salt and pepper to taste

Directions:
1. In a bowl, combine shrimp, lemon zest, lemon juice, minced garlic, chopped cilantro, olive oil, salt, and pepper. Toss until shrimp are well coated.
2. Heat a skillet over medium-high heat. Cook each side of the shrimp for 2-3 minutes until they turn pink and are cooked through.
3. Serve hot as an appetizer or as part of a meal.

Nutritional Value (per serving):
Calories: 160 | Carbs: 2g |
Protein: 20g | Fat: 9g | Fiber: 0g

Thai Inspired Tuna Bowl

Preparation Time: 15 minutes
Cooking Time: 10 minutes
Servings: 2

Ingredients:
- 2 tuna steaks
- 1 tablespoon soy sauce
- 1 tablespoon sesame oil
- 1 teaspoon honey
- 1 clove garlic, minced
- 2 cups cooked rice
- 1 cup mixed vegetables (snap peas, bell peppers, carrots)
- 2 tablespoons chopped peanuts
- Lime wedges for garnish

Directions:
1. In a bowl, mix soy sauce, sesame oil, honey, and minced garlic. Marinate tuna steaks in this mixture for 10 minutes.
2. Heat a grill or skillet over medium-high heat. Cook the tuna steaks for 2-3 minutes per side for medium-rare or until desired doneness. Remove from heat and set aside.

3. In the same skillet, stir-fry mixed vegetables until tender-crisp.

4. Assemble bowls: divide cooked rice among bowls, top with stir-fried vegetables, sliced tuna steaks, and chopped peanuts.

5. Garnish with lime wedges and serve.

Nutritional Value (per serving):
Calories: 450 | Carbs: 45g
Protein: 35g | Fat: 15g | Fiber: 5g

Mediterranean Style Lentil Rice

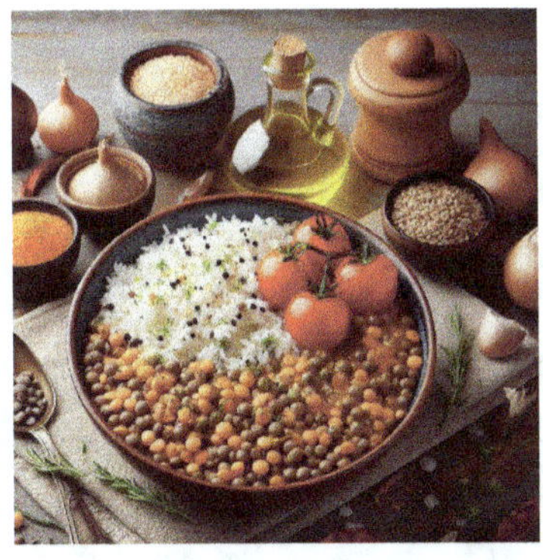

Preparation Time: 10 minutes
Cooking Time: 30 minutes
Servings: 4

Ingredients:
- 1 cup green or brown lentils, rinsed
- 1 cup rice
- 4 cups vegetable broth
- 2 tablespoons olive oil
- 1 onion, finely chopped
- 2 cloves garlic, minced
- 1 teaspoon cumin
- 1 teaspoon paprika
- Salt and pepper to taste
- Chopped parsley for garnish

Directions:

1. In a pot, heat olive oil over medium heat. Add chopped onion and minced garlic. Sauté until softened.

2. Stir in cumin, paprika, salt, and pepper. Cook for another minute.

3. Add lentils and rice to the pot. Stir to coat with the spices.

4. Pour in vegetable broth. Bring to a boil, then reduce heat, cover, and simmer for 20-25 minutes until lentils and rice are cooked and the liquid is absorbed.

5. Fluff with a fork, garnish with chopped parsley, and serve.

Nutritional Value (per serving):
Calories: 320 | Carbs: 55g
Protein: 15g | Fat: 5g | Fiber: 10g

Sautéed Italian Cannellini Beans

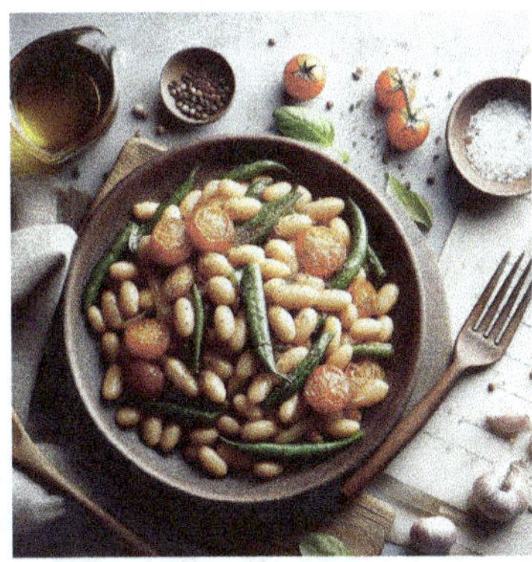

Preparation Time: 10 minutes
Cooking Time: 15 minutes
Servings: 4

Ingredients:
- 2 cans cannellini beans, drained and rinsed
- 2 tablespoons olive oil
- 2 cloves garlic, minced
- 1 teaspoon dried oregano
- 1 teaspoon dried basil
- 1/4 teaspoon red pepper flakes
- Salt and pepper to taste
- Chopped fresh parsley for garnish

Directions:

1. In a skillet set over medium heat, warm the olive oil. Add the minced garlic and cook it until it becomes fragrant.

2. Add cannellini beans, dried oregano, dried basil, red pepper flakes, salt, and pepper. Stir well to combine.

3. Cook for 10-12 minutes, stirring occasionally, until the beans are heated through and flavors meld.

4. Garnish with chopped fresh parsley before serving.

Nutritional Value (per serving):
Calories: 220 | Carbs: 30g |
Protein: 10g | Fat: 7g | Fiber: 8g

Fresh Caprese Pasta Salad

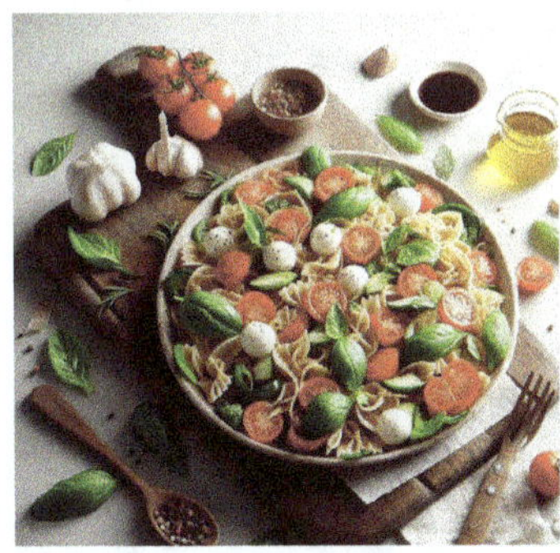

Preparation Time: 15 minutes
Cooking Time: 10 minutes
Servings: 4

Ingredients:
- 8 ounces pasta (penne, fusilli, etc.), cooked according to package instructions
- 2 cups cherry tomatoes, halved
- 1 cup fresh mozzarella, diced
- 1/4 cup fresh basil leaves, chopped
- 2 tablespoons balsamic vinegar
- 3 tablespoons olive oil
- Salt and pepper to taste

Directions:
1. In a large bowl, combine cooked pasta, cherry tomatoes, fresh mozzarella, and chopped basil leaves.
2. Combine the olive oil, salt, pepper, and balsamic vinegar in a small bowl.

3. Pour the dressing over the pasta mixture and toss gently to coat.

4. Serve immediately or refrigerate for a couple of hours before serving to let the flavors meld.

Nutritional Value (per serving):
Calories: 350 | Carbs: 35g |
Protein: 12g | Fat: 18g | Fiber: 3g

Grape-Infused Wild Rice

Preparation Time: 10 minutes
Cooking Time: 45 minutes
Servings: 4

Ingredients:
- 1 cup wild rice
- 2 cups chicken or vegetable broth
- 1 cup seedless grapes, halved
- 1/4 cup chopped pecans or almonds
- 2 tablespoons olive oil
- 2 tablespoons balsamic vinegar
- Salt and pepper to taste
- Chopped parsley for garnish (optional)

Directions:
1. Rinse wild rice under cold water. Heat the broth in a saucepan until it boils. Add wild rice, reduce heat to low, cover, and simmer for 40-45 minutes or until rice is tender and liquid is absorbed.
2. Warm up the olive oil in a pan over medium heat. Add grapes and cook for 2-3 minutes until slightly softened.
3. Add cooked wild rice to the skillet with grapes. Stir in chopped pecans or almonds.

4. Drizzle balsamic vinegar over the rice and grape mixture. Season with salt and pepper to taste. Toss gently to combine.

5. Garnish with chopped parsley before serving.

Nutritional Value (per serving):
Calories: 280 | Carbs: 40g |
Protein: 6g | Fat: 11g | Fiber: 3g

Instant Pot Salmon Poach

Preparation Time: 5 minutes
Cooking Time: 5 minutes (plus time to come to pressure and release pressure)
Servings: 2

Ingredients:
- 2 salmon fillets
- 1 cup water or fish stock
- 2 slices lemon
- Fresh dill for garnish (optional)
- Salt and pepper to taste

Directions:
1. Sprinkle some salt and pepper on the salmon fillets.
2. Pour water or fish stock into the Instant Pot. Place the trivet inside.
3. Lay lemon slices on the trivet and place the seasoned salmon fillets on top.
4. Close the lid, set the valve to the sealing position, and cook on high pressure for 3-4 minutes (depending on thickness).
5. Once done, perform a quick pressure release.

6. Carefully remove the salmon using tongs. Top with freshly chopped dill if preferred and serve hot.

Nutritional Value (per serving):
Calories: 300 | Carbs: 0g |
Protein: 30g | Fat: 20g | Fiber: 0g

Chapter 6: Desserts/Snacks

Savory Zucchini Bites

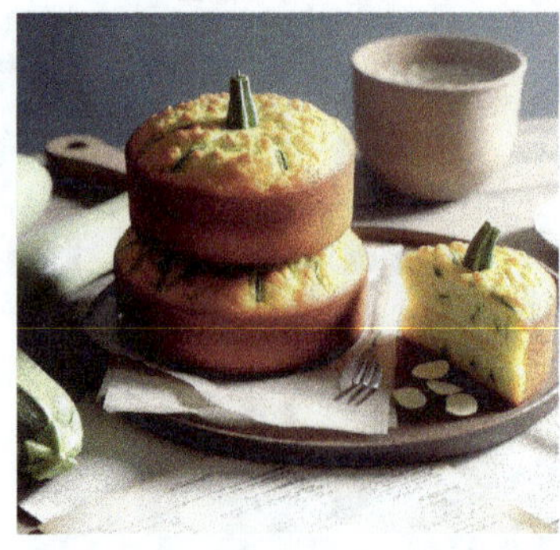

Preparation Time: 15 minutes
Cooking Time: 15 minutes
Servings: 4

Ingredients:
- 2 cups grated zucchini
- 1 egg
- 1/4 cup grated Parmesan cheese
- 1/4 cup breadcrumbs
- 2 tablespoons chopped fresh parsley
- 1 clove garlic, minced
- Salt and pepper to taste
- Olive oil for frying

Directions:
1. Place grated zucchini in a clean kitchen towel or cheesecloth and squeeze out excess moisture.
2. In a bowl, combine grated zucchini, egg, Parmesan cheese, breadcrumbs, chopped parsley,

minced garlic, salt, and pepper. Mix until well combined.

3. In a pan over medium heat, warm the olive oil.

4. Form the zucchini mixture into small patties and gently place them in the skillet.

5. Cook for 3-4 minutes per side until golden brown and cooked through.

6. Remove from the skillet and place on a paper towel-lined plate to absorb excess oil.

7. Serve hot as a snack.

Nutritional Value (per serving):
Calories: 90 | Carbs: 7g |
Protein: 5g | Fat: 5g | Fiber: 2g

Ricotta Fig Toast

Prep Time: 5 minutes | Cooking Time: 5 minutes | Servings: 2

Ingredients:
- 4 slices whole grain bread, toasted
- 1/2 cup ricotta cheese
- 4 fresh figs, sliced
- Honey for drizzling
- Chopped pistachios for garnish (optional)

Directions:

1. Spread ricotta cheese over the toasted bread slices.

2. Arrange sliced figs on top of the ricotta.

3. Drizzle honey over the figs.

4. Garnish with chopped pistachios if desired.

5. Serve immediately as a delicious breakfast or snack.

Nutritional Value (per serving):
Calories: 250 | Carbs: 35g |
Protein: 10g | Fat: 8g | Fiber: 5g

Crunchy Quinoa Snack

Preparation Time: 10 minutes
Cooking Time: 25 minutes
Servings: 8

Ingredients:
- 2 cups cooked quinoa
- 1 cup old-fashioned oats
- ½ cup finely chopped nuts (pecans, almonds, etc.).
- 1/4 cup maple syrup or honey
- 2 tablespoons coconut oil, melted
- 1 teaspoon ground cinnamon
- 1/2 teaspoon vanilla extract
- 1/2 cup dried fruits (cranberries, raisins, etc.)

Directions:
1. Preheat oven to 325°F (160°C). Use parchment paper to line a baking sheet.
2. In a large bowl, combine cooked quinoa, oats, chopped nuts, maple syrup or honey, melted coconut oil, ground cinnamon, and vanilla extract. Mix until well combined.
3. Evenly spread the mixture over the baking sheet that has been prepared.

4. Bake for 20-25 minutes, stirring occasionally, until golden brown and crunchy.

5. Take it out of the oven and allow it to cool fully.

6. Once cooled, stir in dried fruits and store in an airtight container.

Nutritional Value (per serving - 1/2 cup):
Calories: 180 | Carbs: 25g |
Protein: 5g | Fat: 7g | Fiber: 4g

Tart Berry Rhubarb Cobbler

Preparation Time: 20 minutes
Cooking Time: 45 minutes
Servings: 6

Ingredients:
- 4 cups mixed berries (strawberries, blueberries, raspberries)
- 2 cups rhubarb, diced
- 1/2 cup granulated sugar
- 1 tablespoon cornstarch
- 1 cup all-purpose flour
- 1/4 cup granulated sugar (for topping)
- 1 teaspoon baking powder
- 1/4 teaspoon salt
- 1/2 cup cold unsalted butter, diced
- 1/4 cup milk
- Vanilla ice cream for serving (optional)

Directions:
1. Preheat oven to 375°F (190°C).
2. In a bowl, combine mixed berries, diced rhubarb, granulated sugar, and cornstarch. Mix until the fruits are coated evenly. Spoon the mixture into a baking dish.

3. In another bowl, whisk together flour, 1/4 cup sugar, baking powder, and salt.

4. Add cold diced butter to the flour mixture and use your fingers to rub the butter into the flour until it resembles coarse crumbs.

5. Stir in milk until just combined, forming a dough.

6. Drop spoonfuls of the dough over the fruit mixture in the baking dish.

7. Bake for 40-45 minutes or until the top is golden brown and the fruit is bubbling.

8. Before serving, let it cool for a few minutes.

9. If preferred, serve warm with a scoop of vanilla ice cream.

Nutritional Value (per serving):
Calories: 320 | Carbs: 50g |
Protein: 3g | Fat: 13g | Fiber: 5g

Creamy Yogurt Dip

Preparation Time: 5 minutes | Servings: 4

Ingredients:
- 1 cup Greek yogurt
- 1 tablespoon fresh dill, chopped
- 1 tablespoon fresh parsley, chopped
- 1 clove garlic, minced
- Salt and pepper to taste

Directions:
1. In a bowl, combine Greek yogurt, chopped fresh dill, chopped fresh parsley, minced garlic, salt, and pepper. Mix well.
2. Adjust seasoning according to taste preference.
3. Refrigerate for at least 30 minutes before serving to allow flavors to meld.
4. Serve chilled with fresh vegetables, crackers, or chips.

Nutritional Value (per serving):
Calories: 50 | Carbs: 4g |
Protein: 6g | Fat: 1g | Fiber: 0g

Classic Ambrosia Salad

Preparation Time: 15 minutes
Chilling Time: 2 hours
Servings: 6-8

Ingredients:
- 2 cups mandarin oranges (fresh or canned), drained
- 2 cups fresh or canned pineapple chunks, drained
- 1 cup shredded coconut, (unsweetened or sweetened)
- 1 cup mini marshmallows
- 1 cup sour cream or Greek yogurt
- 1 cup whipped topping or whipped cream
- 1 cup drained and cut maraschino cherries
- 1 cup chopped pecans or walnuts, (if desired)
- Fresh mint leaves for garnish (optional)

Directions:

1. In a large mixing bowl, combine mandarin oranges, pineapple chunks, shredded coconut, mini marshmallows, and maraschino cherries. If using nuts, add them as well.

2. In a separate bowl, mix together sour cream or Greek yogurt with whipped topping or whipped cream until well combined.

3. Gently fold the creamy mixture into the fruit mixture until everything is evenly coated.

4. Cover the bowl and refrigerate for at least 2 hours, allowing the flavors to meld and the salad to chill.

5. Before serving, garnish with fresh mint leaves if desired.

Nutritional Value (per serving):
Calories: 270 | Carbs: 35g |
Protein: 3g | Fat: 14g | Fiber: 3g

Crispy Fried Anchovies

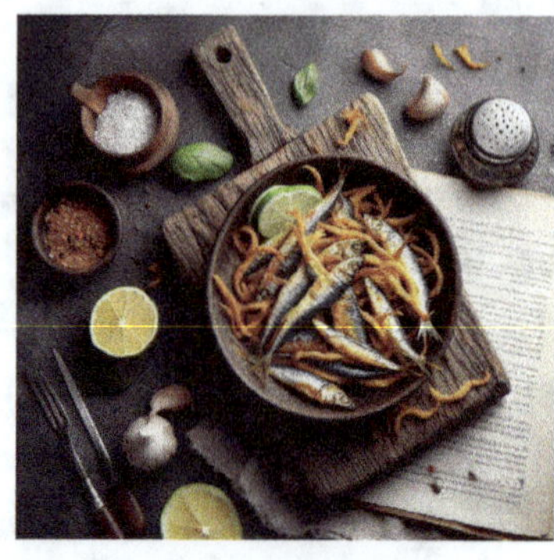

Preparation Time: 15 minutes
Cooking Time: 5 minutes
Servings: 4

Ingredients:
- 1 cup fresh anchovies, cleaned and gutted
- 1/2 cup all-purpose flour
- Salt and pepper to taste
- Vegetable oil for frying
- Lemon wedges for serving

Directions:
1. Rinse the cleaned anchovies and pat dry with paper towels.
2. In a shallow dish, mix flour with salt and pepper.
3. Dredge the anchovies in the seasoned flour, shaking off excess.
4. In a frying pan, heat the vegetable oil over medium-high heat.

5. Until they are crispy and golden brown, fry the anchovies in batches for two to three minutes on each side.

6. Take out from the oil and set on a dish covered with paper towels to absorb extra oil.

7. Serve hot with lemon wedges for squeezing.

Nutritional Value (per serving):
Calories: 150 | Carbs: 10g
Protein: 20g | Fat: 4g | Fiber: 1g

Flavorful Curry Kale Crisps

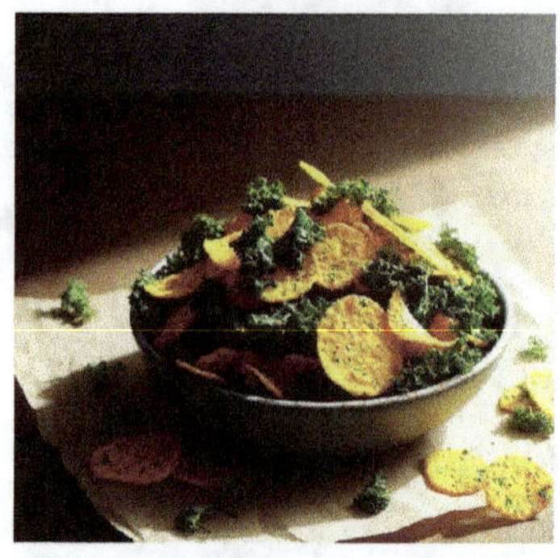

Preparation Time: 10 minutes
Cooking Time: 15-20 minutes
Servings: 4

Ingredients:
- 1 bunch of chopped, bite-sized kale with the stems removed
- 2 tablespoons olive oil
- 1 teaspoon curry powder
- Salt to taste

Directions:
1. Preheat oven to 300°F (150°C). Use a parchment paper to line a baking sheet.
2. In a large bowl, toss the kale pieces with olive oil, curry powder, and salt until evenly coated.
3. Arrange the kale on the prepared baking sheet in a single layer.
4. Bake for 15-20 minutes or until the edges are crisp but not burnt, tossing halfway through.

5. Take them out of the oven and allow them to cool a little before serving.

Nutritional Value (per serving):
Calories: 70 | Carbs: 5g |
Protein: 2g | Fat: 5g | Fiber: 2g

Sweet Potato Bread Toast

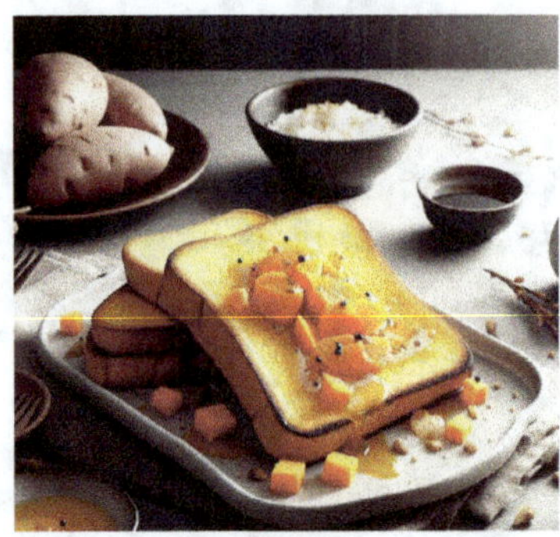

Preparation Time: 5 minutes
Cooking Time: 10-15 minutes
Servings: 2

Ingredients:

- 1 large sweet potato, sliced lengthwise into 1/4-inch thick slices
- Toppings of your choice (avocado, nut butter, eggs, etc.)
- Salt and pepper to taste

Directions:

1. Preheat oven to 400°F (200°C).
2. Place sweet potato slices on a baking sheet lined with parchment paper.
3. Bake for 10-15 minutes or until the slices are tender but not falling apart.
4. Once baked, allow them to cool slightly before adding desired toppings.

5. Add toppings of your choice such as avocado, nut butter, eggs, or any other preferred toppings.

6. Add pepper and salt to taste.

Nutritional Value (per serving - Sweet Potato Slices only):
Calories: 90 | Carbs: 20g
Protein: 2g | Fat: 0g | Fiber: 4g

Raspberry Oat Bars

Preparation Time: 20 minutes
Cooking Time: 30-35 minutes
Servings: 12

Ingredients:
- 1 1/2 cups all-purpose flour
- 1 1/2 cups rolled oats
- 1/2 cup brown sugar
- 1/2 teaspoon baking powder
- 1/4 teaspoon salt
- 1 cup unsalted butter, melted
- 1 cup raspberry jam or preserves

Directions:
1. Preheat oven to 350°F (175°C). Grease a 9x13-inch baking pan.
2. In a large bowl, mix together flour, rolled oats, brown sugar, baking powder, and salt.
3. Add melted butter to the dry ingredients and mix until crumbly.
4. Press two-thirds of the mixture into the bottom of the prepared baking pan.
5. Spread raspberry jam evenly over the pressed mixture.

6. Sprinkle the remaining crumb mixture over the jam layer.

7. Bake for thirty to thirty-five (30-35) minutes, or until golden brown on top.

8. Let it cool fully before slicing it into bars.

Nutritional Value (per serving):
Calories: 250 | Carbs: 35g |
Protein: 2g | Fat: 11g | Fiber: 2g

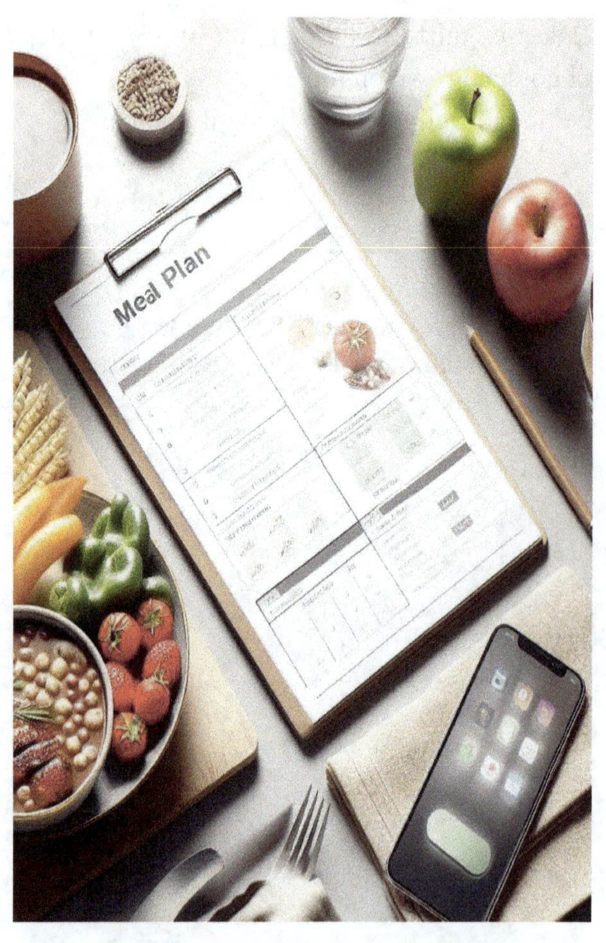

14-Day Meal Plan

Day 1:
Breakfast: Banana-Infused Quinoa Bake
Lunch: Baked Acorn Squash Delight
Dinner: Creamy White Bean Soup
Snack/Dessert: Savory Zucchini Bites

Day 2:
Breakfast: Chia Berry Overnight Oats
Lunch: Spicy Cajun Collard Greens
Dinner: Juicy Lamb Burgers
Snack/Dessert: Ricotta Fig Toast

Day 3:
Breakfast: Hearty Barley Porridge
Lunch: Beef Infusion with Broccoli
Dinner: Quinoa Chicken Fusion Bowls
Snack/Dessert: Crunchy Quinoa Snack

Day 4:
Breakfast: Scrambled Breakfast Tacos
Lunch: Salmon Delight Omelet
Dinner: Citrusy Cilantro Shrimp
Snack/Dessert: Tart Berry Rhubarb Cobbler

Day 5:
Breakfast: Wholesome Feta Egg Bake
Lunch: Flavorful Curry Chicken Salad
Dinner: Thai Inspired Tuna Bowl
Snack/Dessert: Creamy Yogurt Dip

Day 6:
Breakfast: Mixed Farro Salad
Lunch: Savory Swedish Meatballs
Dinner: Mediterranean Style Lentil Rice
Snack/Dessert: Apple Berry Ambrosia

Day 7:
Breakfast: Italian Style Veggie Salad
Lunch: Avocado Infused Shrimp Salad
Dinner: Sautéed Italian Cannellini Beans
Snack/Dessert: Crispy Fried Anchovies

Day 8:
Breakfast: Creamy Spinach Tofu Salad
Lunch: Chicken Lettuce Wraps
Dinner: Grape-Infused Wild Rice
Snack/Dessert: Flavorful Curry Kale Crisps

Day 9:

Breakfast: Crispy Muesli Delight
Lunch: Savory Pork Rice Strips
Dinner: Instant Pot Salmon Poach
Snack/Dessert: Sweet Potato Bread Toast

Day 10:

Breakfast: Bacon Veggie Omelet
Lunch: Mediterranean Seasoned Lamb Chops
Dinner: Fresh Caprese Pasta Salad
Snack/Dessert: Raspberry Oat Bars

Day 11:

Breakfast: Banana-Infused Quinoa Bake
Lunch: Baked Acorn Squash Delight
Dinner: Creamy White Bean Soup
Snack/Dessert: Savory Zucchini Bites

Day 12:

Breakfast: Chia Berry Overnight Oats
Lunch: Spicy Cajun Collard Greens
Dinner: Juicy Lamb Burgers
Snack/Dessert: Ricotta Fig Toast

Day 13:

Breakfast: Hearty Barley Porridge
Lunch: Beef Infusion with Broccoli
Dinner: Quinoa Chicken Fusion Bowls
Snack/Dessert: Crunchy Quinoa Snack

Day 14:

Breakfast: Scrambled Breakfast Tacos
Lunch: Salmon Delight Omelet
Dinner: Citrusy Cilantro Shrimp
Snack/Dessert: Tart Berry Rhubarb Cobbler

This 14-day meal plan offers a variety of delicious and nutritious options for you. Adjust portions as needed and enjoy the flavors!

Conclusion

Alright, folks, here's the lowdown. You've just cracked open the lid on a whole new world of eating—the Pegan way. But guess what? This ain't the end; it's your kick-off into a lifestyle that's all about feeling freakin' fantastic.

You've dabbled in flavors that make your taste buds do a happy dance and stumbled upon meals that fuel you like rocket fuel without the crash. That's the Pegan gig for ya—vibrant, satisfying, and, dare I say, pretty darn tasty.

But hold up, amigo! This ain't a set of strict rules carved in stone. Nah, it's your ticket to figuring out what clicks for your bod. It's your adventure through a jungle of food choices where you're the fearless explorer.

So, big shoutout to you for picking up this book, for diving into a world where health meets real life. Here's to you—may your fridge be stocked with goodness, your meals be a party of flavors, and your journey to feeling awesome be as smooth as your favorite jam.

Listen, it's not about some magic potion; it's about making choices that make you feel like a million bucks. You've got the tools now, buddy. Experiment, mix it up, and savor every bite of this journey.

Thanks for hanging in there with me. Here's wishing you good vibes, epic meals, and a truckload of vitality on your journey ahead. You got this! Cheers to you and your awesome, healthier self!

Weekly Meal Planner

WEEK OF:
....

Sunday
Breakfast..................................
Lunch..................................
Dinner..................................
Snacks..................................

Monday
Breakfast..................................
Lunch..................................
Dinner..................................
Snacks..................................

Tuesday
Breakfast..................................
Lunch..................................
Dinner..................................
Snacks..................................

Wednesday
Breakfast..................................
Lunch..................................
Dinner..................................
Snacks..................................

Thursday
Breakfast..................................
Lunch..................................
Dinner..................................
Snacks..................................

Friday
Breakfast..................................
Lunch..................................
Dinner..................................
Snacks..................................

Saturday
Breakfast..................................
Lunch..................................
Dinner..................................
Snacks..................................

Notes:
____
____
____
____
____

Weekly Meal Planner

WEEK OF: __________
....

Sunday

Breakfast.................................
Lunch.......................................
Dinner......................................
Snacks.....................................

Monday

Breakfast.................................
Lunch.......................................
Dinner......................................
Snacks.....................................

Tuesday

Breakfast.................................
Lunch.......................................
Dinner......................................
Snacks.....................................

Wednesday

Breakfast.................................
Lunch.......................................
Dinner......................................
Snacks.....................................

Thursday

Breakfast.................................
Lunch.......................................
Dinner......................................
Snacks.....................................

Friday

Breakfast.................................
Lunch.......................................
Dinner......................................
Snacks.....................................

Saturday

Breakfast.................................
Lunch.......................................
Dinner......................................
Snacks.....................................

Notes:

____

____

____

____

____

Weekly Meal Planner

WEEK OF: ....

Sunday

Breakfast.....................................
Lunch...
Dinner..
Snacks..

Monday

Breakfast.....................................
Lunch...
Dinner..
Snacks..

Tuesday

Breakfast.....................................
Lunch...
Dinner..
Snacks..

Wednesday

Breakfast.....................................
Lunch...
Dinner..
Snacks..

Thursday

Breakfast.....................................
Lunch...
Dinner..
Snacks..

Friday

Breakfast.....................................
Lunch...
Dinner..
Snacks..

Saturday

Breakfast.....................................
Lunch...
Dinner..
Snacks..

Notes:

____
____
____
____
____

Weekly Meal Planner

WEEK OF:
....

Sunday

Breakfast....................................
Lunch...
Dinner.......................................
Snacks.......................................

Monday

Breakfast....................................
Lunch...
Dinner.......................................
Snacks.......................................

Tuesday

Breakfast....................................
Lunch...
Dinner.......................................
Snacks.......................................

Wednesday

Breakfast....................................
Lunch...
Dinner.......................................
Snacks.......................................

Thursday

Breakfast....................................
Lunch...
Dinner.......................................
Snacks.......................................

Friday

Breakfast....................................
Lunch...
Dinner.......................................
Snacks.......................................

Saturday

Breakfast....................................
Lunch...
Dinner.......................................
Snacks.......................................

Notes:

____

____

____

____

____

Weekly Meal Planner

WEEK OF:
....

Sunday

Breakfast............................
Lunch............................
Dinner............................
Snacks............................

Monday

Breakfast............................
Lunch............................
Dinner............................
Snacks............................

Tuesday

Breakfast............................
Lunch............................
Dinner............................
Snacks............................

Wednesday

Breakfast............................
Lunch............................
Dinner............................
Snacks............................

Thursday

Breakfast............................
Lunch............................
Dinner............................
Snacks............................

Friday

Breakfast............................
Lunch............................
Dinner............................
Snacks............................

Saturday

Breakfast............................
Lunch............................
Dinner............................
Snacks............................

Notes:

____

____

____

____

Weekly Meal Planner

WEEK OF:
....

Sunday
Breakfast...................................
Lunch......................................
Dinner.....................................
Snacks.....................................

Monday
Breakfast...................................
Lunch......................................
Dinner.....................................
Snacks.....................................

Tuesday
Breakfast...................................
Lunch......................................
Dinner.....................................
Snacks.....................................

Wednesday
Breakfast...................................
Lunch......................................
Dinner.....................................
Snacks.....................................

Thursday
Breakfast...................................
Lunch......................................
Dinner.....................................
Snacks.....................................

Friday
Breakfast...................................
Lunch......................................
Dinner.....................................
Snacks.....................................

Saturday
Breakfast...................................
Lunch......................................
Dinner.....................................
Snacks.....................................

Notes:
____
____
____
____
____

Weekly Meal Planner

WEEK OF:

Sunday

Breakfast............................
Lunch..................................
Dinner................................
Snacks...............................

Monday

Breakfast............................
Lunch..................................
Dinner................................
Snacks...............................

Tuesday

Breakfast............................
Lunch..................................
Dinner................................
Snacks...............................

Wednesday

Breakfast............................
Lunch..................................
Dinner................................
Snacks...............................

Thursday

Breakfast............................
Lunch..................................
Dinner................................
Snacks...............................

Friday

Breakfast............................
Lunch..................................
Dinner................................
Snacks...............................

Saturday

Breakfast............................
Lunch..................................
Dinner................................
Snacks...............................

Notes:

Weekly Meal Planner

WEEK OF: ....

Sunday

Breakfast.......................
Lunch............................
Dinner...........................
Snacks..........................

Monday

Breakfast.......................
Lunch............................
Dinner...........................
Snacks..........................

Tuesday

Breakfast.......................
Lunch............................
Dinner...........................
Snacks..........................

Wednesday

Breakfast.......................
Lunch............................
Dinner...........................
Snacks..........................

Thursday

Breakfast.......................
Lunch............................
Dinner...........................
Snacks..........................

Friday

Breakfast.......................
Lunch............................
Dinner...........................
Snacks..........................

Saturday

Breakfast.......................
Lunch............................
Dinner...........................
Snacks..........................

Notes:

____
____
____
____
____

Weekly Meal Planner

WEEK OF: ....

Sunday

Breakfast.............................
Lunch....................................
Dinner...................................
Snacks..................................

Monday

Breakfast.............................
Lunch....................................
Dinner...................................
Snacks..................................

Tuesday

Breakfast.............................
Lunch....................................
Dinner...................................
Snacks..................................

Wednesday

Breakfast.............................
Lunch....................................
Dinner...................................
Snacks..................................

Thursday

Breakfast.............................
Lunch....................................
Dinner...................................
Snacks..................................

Friday

Breakfast.............................
Lunch....................................
Dinner...................................
Snacks..................................

Saturday

Breakfast.............................
Lunch....................................
Dinner...................................
Snacks..................................

Notes:
____
____
____
____
____

Weekly Meal Planner

WEEK OF:
....

Sunday

Breakfast...
Lunch..
Dinner..
Snacks...

Monday

Breakfast...
Lunch..
Dinner..
Snacks...

Tuesday

Breakfast...
Lunch..
Dinner..
Snacks...

Wednesday

Breakfast...
Lunch..
Dinner..
Snacks...

Thursday

Breakfast...
Lunch..
Dinner..
Snacks...

Friday

Breakfast...
Lunch..
Dinner..
Snacks...

Saturday

Breakfast...
Lunch..
Dinner..
Snacks...

Notes:

____

____

____

____

Weekly Meal Planner

WEEK OF:
....

Sunday

Breakfast.....................................
Lunch...
Dinner..
Snacks...

Monday

Breakfast.....................................
Lunch...
Dinner..
Snacks...

Tuesday

Breakfast.....................................
Lunch...
Dinner..
Snacks...

Wednesday

Breakfast.....................................
Lunch...
Dinner..
Snacks...

Thursday

Breakfast.....................................
Lunch...
Dinner..
Snacks...

Friday

Breakfast.....................................
Lunch...
Dinner..
Snacks...

Saturday

Breakfast.....................................
Lunch...
Dinner..
Snacks...

Notes:

____

____

____

____

____

Weekly Meal Planner

WEEK OF:
....

Sunday

Breakfast........................
Lunch........................
Dinner........................
Snacks........................

Monday

Breakfast........................
Lunch........................
Dinner........................
Snacks........................

Tuesday

Breakfast........................
Lunch........................
Dinner........................
Snacks........................

Wednesday

Breakfast........................
Lunch........................
Dinner........................
Snacks........................

Thursday

Breakfast........................
Lunch........................
Dinner........................
Snacks........................

Friday

Breakfast........................
Lunch........................
Dinner........................
Snacks........................

Saturday

Breakfast........................
Lunch........................
Dinner........................
Snacks........................

Notes:

____

____

____

____

Weekly Meal Planner

WEEK OF: ....

Sunday

Breakfast.............................
Lunch.................................
Dinner................................
Snacks................................

Monday

Breakfast.............................
Lunch.................................
Dinner................................
Snacks................................

Tuesday

Breakfast.............................
Lunch.................................
Dinner................................
Snacks................................

Wednesday

Breakfast.............................
Lunch.................................
Dinner................................
Snacks................................

Thursday

Breakfast.............................
Lunch.................................
Dinner................................
Snacks................................

Friday

Breakfast.............................
Lunch.................................
Dinner................................
Snacks................................

Saturday

Breakfast.............................
Lunch.................................
Dinner................................
Snacks................................

Notes:

Weekly Meal Planner

WEEK OF:
....

Sunday

Breakfast......................................
Lunch..
Dinner...
Snacks...

Monday

Breakfast......................................
Lunch..
Dinner...
Snacks...

Tuesday

Breakfast......................................
Lunch..
Dinner...
Snacks...

Wednesday

Breakfast......................................
Lunch..
Dinner...
Snacks...

Thursday

Breakfast......................................
Lunch..
Dinner...
Snacks...

Friday

Breakfast......................................
Lunch..
Dinner...
Snacks...

Saturday

Breakfast......................................
Lunch..
Dinner...
Snacks...

Notes:

____

____

____

____

Weekly Meal Planner

WEEK OF: ....

Sunday

Breakfast.................................
Lunch.......................................
Dinner......................................
Snacks.....................................

Monday

Breakfast.................................
Lunch.......................................
Dinner......................................
Snacks.....................................

Tuesday

Breakfast.................................
Lunch.......................................
Dinner......................................
Snacks.....................................

Wednesday

Breakfast.................................
Lunch.......................................
Dinner......................................
Snacks.....................................

Thursday

Breakfast.................................
Lunch.......................................
Dinner......................................
Snacks.....................................

Friday

Breakfast.................................
Lunch.......................................
Dinner......................................
Snacks.....................................

Saturday

Breakfast.................................
Lunch.......................................
Dinner......................................
Snacks.....................................

Notes:

____

____

____

____

Weekly Meal Planner

WEEK OF: ....

Sunday

Breakfast..............................
Lunch.....................................
Dinner...................................
Snacks..................................

Monday

Breakfast..............................
Lunch.....................................
Dinner...................................
Snacks..................................

Tuesday

Breakfast..............................
Lunch.....................................
Dinner...................................
Snacks..................................

Wednesday

Breakfast..............................
Lunch.....................................
Dinner...................................
Snacks..................................

Thursday

Breakfast..............................
Lunch.....................................
Dinner...................................
Snacks..................................

Friday

Breakfast..............................
Lunch.....................................
Dinner...................................
Snacks..................................

Saturday

Breakfast..............................
Lunch.....................................
Dinner...................................
Snacks..................................

Notes:

____

____

____

____

____

Weekly Meal Planner

WEEK OF:
....

Sunday

Breakfast.................................
Lunch.....................................
Dinner....................................
Snacks...................................

Monday

Breakfast.................................
Lunch.....................................
Dinner....................................
Snacks...................................

Tuesday

Breakfast.................................
Lunch.....................................
Dinner....................................
Snacks...................................

Wednesday

Breakfast.................................
Lunch.....................................
Dinner....................................
Snacks...................................

Thursday

Breakfast.................................
Lunch.....................................
Dinner....................................
Snacks...................................

Friday

Breakfast.................................
Lunch.....................................
Dinner....................................
Snacks...................................

Saturday

Breakfast.................................
Lunch.....................................
Dinner....................................
Snacks...................................

Notes:

____

____

____

____

____

Weekly Meal Planner

WEEK OF: ....

Sunday

Breakfast...............................
Lunch...............................
Dinner...............................
Snacks...............................

Monday

Breakfast...............................
Lunch...............................
Dinner...............................
Snacks...............................

Tuesday

Breakfast...............................
Lunch...............................
Dinner...............................
Snacks...............................

Wednesday

Breakfast...............................
Lunch...............................
Dinner...............................
Snacks...............................

Thursday

Breakfast...............................
Lunch...............................
Dinner...............................
Snacks...............................

Friday

Breakfast...............................
Lunch...............................
Dinner...............................
Snacks...............................

Saturday

Breakfast...............................
Lunch...............................
Dinner...............................
Snacks...............................

Notes:

____
____
____
____
____

WEEK OF:
....

Sunday	**Monday**
Breakfast..........................	Breakfast..........................
Lunch..........................	Lunch..........................
Dinner..........................	Dinner..........................
Snacks..........................	Snacks..........................
Tuesday	**Wednesday**
Breakfast..........................	Breakfast..........................
Lunch..........................	Lunch..........................
Dinner..........................	Dinner..........................
Snacks..........................	Snacks..........................
Thursday	**Friday**
Breakfast..........................	Breakfast..........................
Lunch..........................	Lunch..........................
Dinner..........................	Dinner..........................
Snacks..........................	Snacks..........................
Saturday	Notes:
Breakfast..........................	
Lunch..........................	
Dinner..........................	
Snacks..........................	

WEEK OF:
....

Sunday	Monday
Breakfast...........................	Breakfast...........................
Lunch................................	Lunch................................
Dinner...............................	Dinner...............................
Snacks...............................	Snacks...............................

Tuesday	Wednesday
Breakfast...........................	Breakfast...........................
Lunch................................	Lunch................................
Dinner...............................	Dinner...............................
Snacks...............................	Snacks...............................

Thursday	Friday
Breakfast...........................	Breakfast...........................
Lunch................................	Lunch................................
Dinner...............................	Dinner...............................
Snacks...............................	Snacks...............................

Saturday	Notes:
Breakfast...........................	__________________
Lunch................................	__________________
Dinner...............................	__________________
Snacks...............................	__________________

Weekly Meal Planner

WEEK OF:
....

Sunday

Breakfast..................................
Lunch.......................................
Dinner......................................
Snacks......................................

Monday

Breakfast..................................
Lunch.......................................
Dinner......................................
Snacks......................................

Tuesday

Breakfast..................................
Lunch.......................................
Dinner......................................
Snacks......................................

Wednesday

Breakfast..................................
Lunch.......................................
Dinner......................................
Snacks......................................

Thursday

Breakfast..................................
Lunch.......................................
Dinner......................................
Snacks......................................

Friday

Breakfast..................................
Lunch.......................................
Dinner......................................
Snacks......................................

Saturday

Breakfast..................................
Lunch.......................................
Dinner......................................
Snacks......................................

Notes:

____

____

____

____

____